Contents

Introduction

The 7-Day Color Diet is a clever way to get you to eat fruits and vegetables. It uses the principles from the National Cancer Institute's 2002 "Savor the Spectrum" program, which promotes healthy eating by suggesting that people eat five to nine servings of fruit and vegetables a day. Inspired by the concept of colorful foods being healthy, artist Mindy Weisel, along with her two daughters, wrote the book "The 7-Day Color Diet" in 2003.

What is a 7-Day Color Diet?

The 7-Day Color Diet is not a new idea, but it's newly popular. The idea behind it is that colourful vegetables and fruit contain specific micronutrients that support your health and combat biological stress with antioxidants and anti-inflammatory molecules.

This type of biological stress affects your body at a cellular level - you probably know it as "oxidative stress", which is caused by free radicals. Fortunately, the antioxidants in rainbow diet foods help the body to neutralise free radicals and stop them from

damaging your cells.

Free radicals are generated by your

metabolism (the sum of life-giving chemical

reactions inside your cells) and your

environment. Here are some common

sources of free radicals in everyday life:

- Mitochondria

- Inflammation

- Exercise

- Cigarette smoke and air pollutants

- Pesticides, radiation, industrial

  solvents

The rainbow diet nutrients don't act directly on free radicals. Instead, they prompt your body's natural antioxidant mechanisms, which increases your natural ability to reduce oxidative stress. It also has a few other great benefits too.

Plant foods are full of fibre, and fibre is what keeps your digestive system running optimally. Plus, fibre and other plant nutrients are prebiotics: food molecules for your gut bacteria that also help keep you healthy.

Mindy is an artist and author of 7-Day Color Diet (which this book is a follow up to), Carolyn is a licensed nutritionist and Jessica is an esthecian (a person who specializes in the beautification of the skin). Each of the authors contribute to the book Mindy writes about how to do the diet.

Mindy originally became interested in using the colour of food as a dietary aid, when she was doing graduate work as an artist, she asked an art student what she did to stay slim, the student replied that

She was only eating foods that were

orange-cantaloupe, carrots, cheddar cheese

and so on

She doesn't say that the student was

drinking her own push, but she probably

did, it's orangish and those artist types are

all mental.

This caught Mindy's imagination and she

decided to concentrate on the colours of

food and not the calories or carbohydrate

content, etc.

Soon I was imagining days of focusing only

on blue foods, red foods and so on

Eh? Blue foods? Can't think of a single one,

no wonder she lost weight.

The crux of the diet is that white foods form

the base of the diet (day 1 is white), then

every subsequent day you add different

colour to the diet e.g. Day 3 is a green day,

so you eat stuff from the white day and add

in green foods. Day 4 is an orange day so

you eat everything from the white day and

add in orange foods.

Colors of Food

Different colored foods have different nutritional benefits. The 7-Day Color Diet provides recipes using nutritional foods based on scientific evidence. Each day of the week is devoted to a specific color. Day one is white, day two is red, day three is green, day four is orange, day five is purple, day six is yellow, and on day seven you eat the rainbow of colors. If you follow and stick with the diet, you should lose weight, maintain a healthy weight and maybe even improve your complexion.

White, Red and Green

Dr. Julie Garden-Robinson, a food and
nutrition specialist, explains the particular
benefits of each food color group in a
pamphlet put out by the North Dakota State
University Extension Service. Foods in day
one's white group are bananas, cauliflower,
garlic, ginger, jicama, mushrooms, onions
and potatoes. White foods contain
anthoxanthins, which may lower blood
pressure and cholesterol. Foods in day
two's red group are red apples, beets,
cherries, pink grapefruit, red grapes, red
peppers, red potatoes, strawberries,

tomatoes and watermelon. Red foods

contain lycopene, which may reduce

prostate cancer risk. Spaghetti sauce made

with tomatoes, for example, is an excellent

way for your body to absorb lycopene.

Foods in day three's green group are green

apples, artichokes, avocados, asparagus,

broccoli, green beans, cucumbers, green

grapes, peas, lettuce, limes, green pepper,

spinach and zucchini. Green foods contain

chlorophyll. Some contain lutein, which

combined with zeaxanthin -- found in

grapes, corn, red pepper, egg yolks and

oranges -- may reduce cataracts. Other green vegetables can help protect against some forms of cancer.

WHITE

White foods can save you from next day headaches. White foods like Milk, Oats, Yogurt, Cauliflower, Garlic, Onions, and Mushrooms are filled with energy in the form of allicin. They have medicinal properties like lowering cholesterol and blood pressure symptoms. The fruits like bananas and Turnips are the power bank for Potassium and Magnesium. They protect our body from bacterial infections.

Another major property of white foods is

'probiotics', which promotes digestive and

immune power.

Fruits and veggies

- cauliflower

- garlic

- leeks

- onions

- mushrooms

- daikon radish

- parsnips

- white potatoes

Main phytonutrients

anthoxanthins (flavonols, flavones), allicin

Main vitamins and minerals

- fiber

- folate

- magnesium

- manganese

- potassium

- vitamin B6

- vitamin K1

Health benefits

- anti-inflammatory

- antioxidant

- may lower your risk of colon and other cancers

- may benefit heart health

RED

Red is the color of the Sun, so it is for Sunday. Red is the color of Heart, so it is good for Heart health. Red is a color of blood, so it is essential for blood. In general, red fruits and vegetables are always high in antioxidant properties, which have the

property like guarding us against cancer.

Red fruits and vegetables like Tomatoes,

Apples, Beets, and Cherries are rich in

antioxidants and fight radicals produced in

the tissue molecules.

Fruits and veggies

- tomatoes

- tomato paste

- tomato sauce

- watermelon

- pink guava

- grapefruit

Main phytonutrients

lycopene (from the vitamin A family)

Main vitamins and minerals

- folate

- potassium

- vitamin A (lycopene)

- vitamin C

- vitamin K1

Health benefits

- anti-inflammatory

- antioxidant

- may benefit heart health

- may reduce sun-related skin damage

- may lower your risk of certain cancers

GREEN

Green is a color of nature; hence it is healthy for the body. Green is a color of peace; hence it is good for body heat and mental problems. The Green color of the food comes from the 'chlorophyll'. It is because of the photosynthesis process by the plant. Green foods are mostly leafy foods like spinach, cabbage, parsley, Broccoli etc., Green foods are rich in potassium, Vitamin k, folic acid etc., and they are the super food for humans. Green fruits like green apple, cucumber, Kiwi are called summer fruits because they reduce body temperature and helps to control heat stroke, stress, insomnia etc.

Fruits and veggies

- spinach
- kale
- broccoli
- avocados
- asparagus
- green cabbage

- Brussels sprouts

- green herbs

Main phytonutrients

- Leafy greens: chlorophyll and carotenoids

- Cruciferous greens (e.g., broccoli, cabbage): indoles, isothiocyanates, glucosinolates

Main vitamins and minerals

- fiber

- folate

- magnesium

- potassium

- vitamin A (beta carotene)

- vitamin K1

Health benefits

- anti-inflammatory

- antioxidant

- cruciferous veggies, in particular, may

  lower your risk of cancer and heart

  disease

Orange, Purple and Yellow

Foods in day four's orange group and in day

six's yellow group are yellow apples,

apricots, butternut squash, carrots,

grapefruit, lemons, nectarines, mangoes,

oranges, peaches, pears, yellow peppers,

pineapple, corn, sweet potatoes and

tangerines. Orange/yellow foods contain

carotenoids, which help with eye health,

reduce the risk of some cancers, help

prevent heart disease and improve your

immune system. Foods in day five's purple

group are blackberries, blueberries, plums,

eggplant, figs, purple grapes, prunes and

raisins. Purple foods contain anthocyanins,

which are antioxidants that protect your

cells from damage. Blueberries, in particular, can help with memory loss due to aging.

ORANGE

Orange is always a special color for all; it is a color of the eye. Hence Orange-colored fruits and vegetables are essential for our eyes. Orange foods are rich in carotenoids. It is essential for eyesight. Vitamin A is the power bank of orange foods. The orange veggies like carrot, pumpkins, and fruits like orange and papaya are so good for eye vision. Orange foods are also filled with magnesium and vitamin c, which helps to increase sperm counts and reduce birth defects.

Orange vegetables

There's nothing groundbreaking about orange vegetables in the rainbow diet food chart. In fact, you've probably eaten some of them already this week. You can turbocharge your intake with delicious pumpkin soups, roasted sweet potatoes, and spices like turmeric.

- Carrot

- Orange bell pepper

- Pumpkin

- Turmeric

- Sweet potatoes

- Yams

Orange fruits

The rainbow diet food list of orange fruits is
also inspiring and seasonal. Add cantaloupe
and fresh apricots to your diet in summer,
and citrus and persimmon in winter to
boost your body's natural antioxidant
mechanisms.

- Apricots

- Blood orange

- Cantaloupe

- Kumquat

- Mandarine

- Mango

- Nectarine

- Oranges

- Papaya

- Passionfruit

- Peach

- Persimmon

YELLOW

Yellow is the color of brightness, hence it is good for eye and eyesight. Like orange-colored foods, yellow colored foods are also rich in carotenoids or beta-carotenoids. Taking fruits like lemon, Mangoes, Pineapple reduces the body heat during summer. Vegetables like corn, squash, and pumpkins are good fiber foods and help to maintain body weight. Moreover, they contain unsaturated fats which are too good for healthy skin and heart.

Fruits and veggies

- sweet potatoes

- yellow peppers

- bananas

- pineapple

- corn

- Apples (Golden Delicious)

- Asian Pears

- Bananas

- Lemons

- Starfruit

Main phytonutrients

carotenoids (e.g., beta carotene, alpha carotene, beta cryptoxanthin), which belong to the vitamin A family

Main vitamins and minerals

- fiber

- folate

- potassium

- vitamin A (beta carotene)

- vitamin C

Health benefits

- anti-inflammatory

- antioxidant

- may benefit heart health

- supports eye health

- may lower your risk of cancer

PURPLE

Purple is generally called as a girl's favorite

color because naturally they get attracted

towards purple color. Hence, Purple color

fruits and vegetables are the best foods for

menstrual cramps and irregular period's

problems. They too have high antioxidant property and anthocyanin content, which gives the purple color to the fruit or vegetable. The fruits like blueberries, grapes, pomegranates are very rich in anthocyanin content. Figs are rich with calcium content and most recommended for weight loss.

Fruits and veggies

- blueberries

- blackberries

- Concord grapes

- red/purple cabbage

- eggplant

- plums

- elderberries

Main phytonutrients

anthocyanins

Main vitamins and minerals

- fiber

- manganese

- potassium

- vitamin B6

- vitamin C

- vitamin K1

Health benefits

- anti-inflammatory

- antioxidant

- may benefit heart health

- may lower your risk of neurological disorders

- may improve brain function

- may lower your risk of type 2 diabetes

- may lower your risk of certain cancers

If you are disciplined, you can eat a rainbow of colorful foods every day. Make your plate visually pleasing by eating vibrantly colored fresh foods. If you want to give this new way of eating a kick start, follow the day-by-day color suggestions. Even though each day stars one particular color, your diet can still contain variety. For example, on white day, some salads from which to choose are cold cauliflower salad with nonfat yogurt

and Dijon mustard, mushroom and endive

salad with herb vinaigrette or white day

luncheon salad with vinaigrette dressing

that contains white cabbage, low-fat Swiss

cheese, lettuce and an egg. If you prefer

soup, try the Russian mushroom soup on

white day made with chicken stock and

seasoned with caraway seeds, paprika and

dill.

Meal Plan

Day one (White)

Each meal has to have protein in it to keep you feeling full. Fruit, vegetables and complex carbs are all recommended.

Here's the complex carbs that can be added at breakfast or lunch

- 1 slice bread (rye, wheat or pumpernickel

- 1 cup cereal (high fibre – low fat, i.e. oatmeal, All Bran, go Lean, or Bran Flakes)

- 1 English Muffin (whole wheat)

- 1 small whole what pitta bread

- 2 rye crisp crackers, 2 rice cakes, or 3 melba toasts

- 1 cup brown rice

- 1 cup whole wheat pasta

- 1 small baked potato

- 1 ounce oat bran pretzels

Here's the Protein list that you can add (you should have one portion of protein per meal)

- One 4 ounce serving or porting from the recipes in each colour day

- One 4 ounce serving of fish, chicken, turkey or tofu

- 1 cup of cottage chess (low fat)

- 1 cup non-fat or low-fat yoghurt (may also be used in soups, dressing or desserts)

- 1 tablespoon of peanut butter

Here's some White foods that you can add to each meal (or snack)

White fruit:

- White grapefruit

- White Vegetables:

Unlimited amounts of mushrooms, onions, cabbage, cauliflower, endive, bean sprouts, pattypan squash, water chestnuts

 From this point onward, white proteins, complex carbs, fruit and vegetables form the core of your diet but you add fruits, vegetables and protein appropriate for the colour day to each meal (the authors don't list which proteins you can have. here's the ones that I can think of red meat, white/orange/red/yellow fish or white poultry).

Day 2 (Red)

Red Fruits

1 cup strawberries, 1 apple, 1 cup of

raspberries, 1 cup watermelon

 Red Juices

6 ounces tomatoe juice or 6 ounces V-8

juice

Red Vegetables

1 tomato; unlimited amounts of red

cabbed, radishes, pimientos, red peppers

Day 3 (Green)

Green fruits

1 pear, 1 cup of frozen honeydew balls, 1/4

cup green grapes, 1 small green apple

Green vegetables

unlimited amounts of asparagus, broccoli,

brussel sprouts, cucumber, celery, chard,

green beans, lettuce, spinach, courgette

Day 4 (Orange)

Orange fruits

1 orange or 1/2 cup of orange juice, 1/2

cantaloupe, 1 mango, 1 fresh peach or 1/2

cup canned in it's own juice; 1/2/ papaya; 2

fresh apricots or 4 halves canned in their

own juice; 1 tangerine; 1 nectarine

Orange vegetables

Unlimited amounts of carrots

Day 5 (Purple)

Purple Fruits

2 fresh or canned plums, juice pack, 1 cup

blueberries, 1 cup blackberries

Purple vegetables

Unlimited amounts of beets, aubergine ,

purple cabbage

Day 6 (Yellow)

Yellow Fruits

1 banana; 1/2/ cup pineapple, 1 small golden delicious apple, lemons

Yellow vegetables

Unlimited amounts of yellow squash, wax beans? (Eh? What the fuck are wax beans?)

Day 7 (Rainbow)

All the food from the other six colour days.

Recipe

Pumpkin-Date Smoothie

Ingredients

- 1 cup vanilla almond milk (or soy or dairy)

- 1/2 cup pumpkin puree

- 1 banana (frozen is best)

- 1/4 cup dates, softened for a few minutes in hot water

- 1/4 teaspoon pumpkin pie spice

- 1/2 cup cooked white beans

- 1/2 teaspoon vanilla extract

- 1 cup ice cubes

Instructions

1. Blend on high in a blender until
    smooth, about 1 minute. Serves 2.

Pumpkin-Pecan Yogurt Parfait

Ingredients

- 1/2 cup low-fat plain Greek yogurt

- 1/4 cup pumpkin puree

- 2 tablespoons pecans, chopped

- Sprinkle of cinnamon

- Drizzle of maple syrup

- Tiny pinch of kosher salt

Instructions

1. Layer in order into a parfait cup or
    small bowl and enjoy. Serves 1. It's
    great for breakfast, a snack or
    dessert.

Pumpkin Soy Vanilla Latte

Ingredients

- 1 1/2 cups vanilla soy milk divided

- 1/2 cup pumpkin puree

- 1/4 teaspoon pumpkin pie spice

- 2 teaspoons instant espresso powder

Instructions

1. In a blender, mix half the soy milk,
   the pumpkin puree, the pumpkin pie
   spice and the espresso on medium
   until smooth.

2. Fill two glasses with ice.

3. Pour the pumpkin coffee mixture
   over the ice.

4. Top with the remaining vanilla soy
   milk. Add a straw and serve.

Pumpkin Rice Pudding

Ingredients

- 2 cups water

- 1 cup arborio rice

- 3 cups reduced-fat (2%) milk

- 1 cup solid-pack pure pumpkin (not pumpkin pie filling)

- 3/4 cup honey

- 1 teaspoon vanilla extract

- 3/4 teaspoon ground cinnamon, plus more for garnish

- 1/4 teaspoon ground ginger

- 1/4 teaspoon ground nutmeg

- 1/4 teaspoon salt

- 1/3 cup heavy whipping cream, whipped

Directions

1. Preheat the oven to 375F.

2. Bring the water to a boil in an ovenproof 4-quart saucepan. Stir in the rice and cover. Reduce the heat to low and simmer until the rice is nearly cooked, about 20 minutes.

3. In a large bowl, whisk together the milk, pumpkin, honey, vanilla, cinnamon, ginger, nutmeg, and salt.

4. While the rice is still hot, add the pumpkin mixture to the saucepan and stir well to combine. Cover and transfer to the oven.

5. Bake until the liquid has reduced by about a third and the mixture is foamy and bubbling, 45 to 50 minutes.

6. Remove from the oven and stir well to combine all the ingredients. Transfer to a large bowl, then cover and chill in the refrigerator for at least 8 hours or overnight. The

pudding will keep for up to 4 days in
an airtight container in the
refrigerator.

7. Serve with a dollop of whipped cream
    and a sprinkling of cinnamon.

Ingredients

- Vegetable oil cooking spray

Filling

- 1 (13-ounce) jar apricot jam or
  preserves (about 1 1/4 cups)

- 8 dried apricots, chopped into 1/4-

  inch pieces (about 1/3 cup)

Crust

- 1 3/4 cups all-purpose flour

- 1 packed cup light brown sugar

- 1 teaspoon ground cinnamon

- 3/4 teaspoon fine sea salt

- 3/4 teaspoon baking soda

- 1 3/4 cups old-fashioned oats

- 1 cup (4 ounces) coarsely chopped

  walnuts

- 1 cup (2 sticks) unsalted butter,

  melted

- 1 egg, at room temperature, beaten

- 1 teaspoon pure vanilla extract

Directions

1. Put an oven rack in the center of the oven. Preheat the oven to 350 degrees F.

2. Spray a 9 by 13 by 2-inch metal baking dish with vegetable oil cooking spray.

3. Line the bottom and sides of the pan with parchment paper.

4. Spray the parchment paper with vegetable oil cooking spray and set aside.

Filling

1. In a small bowl, mix together the jam and the apricots. Set aside.

Crust

1. In a large bowl, whisk together the flour, sugar, cinnamon, salt and baking soda. Stir in the oats and walnuts. Add the butter, egg and vanilla and stir until incorporated.

2. Using a fork or clean fingers, lightly press half of the crust mixture onto the bottom of the prepared pan.

3. Using a spatula, spread the filling over the crust leaving a 1/2-inch border around the edge of the pan.

4. Cover the filling with the remaining crust mixture and gently press to **flatten.**

5. Bake until light golden, about 30 to 35 minutes. Cool for 1 hour.

6. Cut into bars and store in an airtight container for up to 3 days.

Ingredients

- 1 medium cantaloupe (about 3 pounds)

- 1 medium honeydew (about 3 pounds)

- 1 1/2 pounds thinly sliced prosciutto (about 36 slices)

- 2 bunches fresh chives, blanch 36 and save remaining for garnish

Directions

1. Working with 1 melon at a time, cut in 1/2. Gently scrape out seeds and membrane and discard. Using a melon baller, scoop out rounds from flesh and place in large bowl. Discard skin.

2. Keep the prosciutto loosely covered with plastic wrap to prevent them from drying out as you start to assemble 1 purse at a time. Place 1 melon ball in the center of a prosciutto slice, gather all sides to the

top and secure with a blanched chive.
It may be necessary to overlap a few
pieces of prosciutto in order to
completely wrap the melon ball.

3. Place the finished purse, seam side
down onto a baking sheet and keep
covered. Repeat with remaining
prosciutto and melons.

4. Can make it only up to 2 hours ahead
of time because the salt in the
prosciutto will break down the
melon.

5. Scatter the chives onto a decorative platter. Place prosciutto purses on top and serve.

Carrot Salad

Ingredients

- 6 large carrots, peeled

- 1/4 cup fresh lemon juice

- 2 cloves garlic, finely chopped

- 2 teaspoons ground cumin

- 1/2 teaspoon cayenne pepper

- 1 teaspoon salt, plus more for water

- 1/4 cup olive oil

- 1/4 cup finely chopped flat-leaf

   parsley

Directions

1. Bring a large pot of salted water to a

   boil.

2. Add the whole carrots (cut them in

   half if they don't fit in the pot) and

   cook until just cooked through, about

   8 to 10 minutes.

3. Drain and cut carrots into 1/2-inch

   thick slices.

4. Whisk together the lemon juice,

    garlic, cumin, cayenne, and salt in a

    large bowl.

5. Slowly drizzle in the olive oil until

    emulsified and stir in the parsley.

6.   Add the cooked carrots and toss to

    combine. Serve cold or at room

    temperature.

Mango Salsa

Ingredients

- 1 mango, peeled and diced

- 1/2 cup peeled, diced cucumber

- 1 tablespoon finely chopped jalapeno

- 1/3 cup diced red onion

- 1 tablespoon lime juice

- 1/3 cup roughly chopped cilantro

  leaves

- Salt and pepper

Directions

1. Combine the mango, cucumber,

   jalapeno, red onion, lime juice and

   cilantro leaves and mix well.

2. Season with salt and pepper, to taste.

3.

Honey Roasted Sweet Potatoes

Ingredients

- 2 pounds red-skinned sweet potatoes

- 2 tablespoons olive oil

- 2 tablespoons honey

- 1 teaspoon fresh lemon juice

- 1/2 teaspoon salt

Directions

1. Preheat the oven to 350 degrees F.

2. Peel and cut the sweet potatoes into 1-inch pieces and put in a 9 by 13 baking dish.

3. In a small bowl whisk together olive

    oil, honey and lemon juice. Pour

    mixture over potatoes and toss to

    coat.

4. Sprinkle with the salt, and bake,

    stirring occasionally, for about 1

    hour, until potatoes are tender.

Tomato Crostini

Ingredients

- 6 to 8 Servings

- 2 pounds ripe tomatoes, cored, halved, seeded, chopped into 1-inch-thick slices

- 3 garlic cloves, 2 minced, 1 halved

- Sea salt and freshly ground black pepper

- 3 tablespoons extra-virgin olive plus more for drizzling

- 1tablespoon red wine vinegar

- 1 loaf ciabatta or baguette, cut on a diagonal into 1/3' pieces

- 1/4 cup packed fresh basil leaves, coarsely chopped

Preparation

Step 1

Combine tomatoes and minced garlic in a large bowl. Season generously with salt and pepper. Add 3 Tbsp. oil and vinegar; toss to mix well. Cover and let tomatoes marinate at room temperature, stirring occasionally, for 2–3 hours to allow flavors to develop.

Step 2

Rub one side of toasted bread with cut sides of remaining garlic clove; drizzle bread with oil and cut in half crosswise. Add basil to tomato mixture in bowl and toss well.

Season to taste with salt and pepper.

Arrange crostini on a platter. Spoon some

tomato mixture on top of each crostini.

Mixed Berry Gazpacho with Basil

Ingredients

- 3 cups mixed berries (about 1 lb.); if using strawberries, cut into 1/2' pieces

- 2 tablespoons sugar

- 1 tablespoon fresh orange juice

- 1 teaspoon finely grated lemon zest

- 1 teaspoon lemon juice

- 1 teaspoon fresh lime juice

- 1 sprig basil, torn into pieces, plus

  small leaves for garnish

- Extra-virgin olive oil (for drizzling)

- Freshly ground black pepper

- Vanilla ice cream

Preparation

Step 1

Combine first 6 ingredients and basil sprig

in a medium heatproof bowl; toss to coat.

Cover with plastic wrap. Place over a large

saucepan of simmering water; cook for 10

minutes.

Step 2

Let cool for 15 minutes. Chill until cold,

about 4 hours. DO AHEAD: Berry gazpacho

can be made 1 day ahead. Keep chilled.

Step 3

Divide fruit and juices among bowls; drizzle

with oil, garnish with basil leaves and

pepper, and top with a scoop of ice cream.

Ingredients

SPECIAL EQUIPMENT

- A deep-fry thermometer

Preparation

Step 1

Pour vegetable oil into a small heavy

saucepan to a depth of 1 inch. Prop deep-

fry thermometer in oil so bulb is

submerged; heat oil over medium heat to

350°. Add four 3-inch rosemary sprigs to oil

and fry until crisp and bright green, 10-15

seconds. Transfer to a paper towel-lined

plate; season lightly with kosher salt. Add

10 pitted oil-cured black olives to oil; fry

until bubbling stops, about 4 minutes. Place

on plate with rosemary. Strip rosemary

leaves from sprigs; mince. Chop olives.

Using a small, sharp knife, cut peel and

white pith from 6 blood oranges and 6 Cara

Cara oranges. Cut crosswise into 1/2 inches

rounds; arrange on a platter.

DO AHEAD: Oranges, rosemary, and olives

can be prepared 6 hours ahead. Cover and

chill orange slices. Separately store

rosemary and olives airtight at room temperature.

Step 2

Season oranges lightly with salt and freshly ground black pepper; drizzle with 2 tablespoons extra-virgin olive oil. Sprinkle chopped rosemary and olives over oranges.

Cranberry-Citrus Sorbet

Ingredients

- 3 cups leftover cranberry sauce
- 1 cup fresh orange juice
- 1 /2 cup fresh lemon juice

- 1/4 cup sugar

- 1/4 cup water

- 2 tablespoons grated orange peel

- 1 tablespoon grated lemon peel

Preparation

Step 1

Bring all ingredients to a simmer in a heavy medium pot over medium-high heat. Cook until sugar is dissolved and mixture is heated through, about 5 minutes. Transfer mixture to a 9x13-inch metal baking pan. Place the pan in the freezer. Freeze for 3 hours, stirring with a spoon every hour to break up ice crystals. Scoop mixture into chilled bowls and serve.

Plum and Mascarpone Pie

Ingredients

- 1 pie crust, homemade or store-bought (click for homemade crust recipe)

- 4-5 pounds firm ripe plums (20–25 plums), halved, pitted (with skin)

- 1 1/2 cups plus 2 Tbsp. sugar

- 2 tablespoons fresh lemon juice

- 1 vanilla bean, split lengthwise

- 8 ounces mascarpone

- 1/3 cup crème fraîche

- 2 tablespoons honey

- Whipped cream

Preparation

Step 1

Preheat oven to 350°. Line pie dish with crust; crimp edges. Fully bake pie crust according to recipe or box instructions.

Step 2

Place plums in a large bowl; add 1 1/2 cups sugar and lemon juice. Scrape in seeds from half of vanilla bean; toss to coat. Divide plum mixture between two 13x9x2" glass baking dishes, arranging plums cut side down and overlapping slightly. Roast until juices are bubbling and slightly thickened and plums are tender but not falling apart, 40–60 minutes (cooking time will depend on ripeness of plums). Let cool slightly.

Step 3

Using a slotted spatula, transfer plums to a

rimmed baking sheet. Cover loosely with

plastic wrap; chill. Pour juices in baking

dishes into a small saucepan. Bring to a boil

and simmer until thickened and reduced to

a scant 1/2 cup, 4–5 minutes; set glaze

aside.

Step 4

Combine remaining 2 Tbsp. sugar,

mascarpone, crème fraîche, and honey in a

medium bowl. Scrape in seeds from

remaining half vanilla bean. Using an

electric mixer, beat on high speed until

mixture holds firm peaks (do not overbeat

or mascarpone may curdle).

DO AHEAD: Plums, glaze, and mascarpone

cream can be made 1 day ahead. Cover

separately and chill.

Step 5

Spread mascarpone cream evenly over

bottom of crust. Arrange some chilled plum

halves tightly (but not overlapping) in a

single layer over mascarpone mixture.

Starting at edges of pie crust, arrange

remaining plum halves on top of base layer,

overlapping tightly and forming a spiral to
cover. Pie should dome slightly in the
center.

Step 6

Using a pastry brush, spread some of glaze
over plums (if glaze has firmed up, gently
reheat, adding 1 Tbsp. water and whisking
to blend).

Step 7

Cut pie into slices. Top with whipped cream
and drizzle with more plum syrup.

Tomato and Cheddar Pie

Ingredients

CRUST

- 2 cups all-purpose flour

- 1 1/2 teaspoons baking powder

- 1/2 teaspoon baking soda

- 1/2 teaspoon kosher salt

- 6 tablespoons (3/4 stick) chilled

  unsalted butter, cut into 1/2' cubes

- 3/4 cup buttermilk

- FILLING

- 2 pounds large ripe tomatoes, cored

  and cut into 1/4' slices

- 2 1/2 cups coarsely grated extra-

  sharp cheddar (8-9 ounces)

- 1/4 cup finely grated Parmesan (1/2

  ounce)

- 1 scallion, trimmed, chopped

- 1/2 cup mayonnaise

- 2 tablespoons chopped fresh dill

- 1 tablespoon apple cider vinegar

- 2 teaspoons sugar

- 3/4 teaspoon kosher salt

- 1/2 teaspoon freshly ground black pepper

- 1 1/2 tablespoons cornmeal

Preparation

CRUST

Step 1

Whisk first 4 ingredients in a medium bowl. Using your fingertips, rub in butter until a coarse meal forms and some small lumps remain. Stir in buttermilk and knead gently with your hands until dough forms. Wrap dough in plastic and chill for 1 hour.

FILLING

Step 2

Lay tomatoes in a single layer on a baking

sheet lined with 2 layers of paper towels.

Place another 2 layers of paper towels on

top of tomatoes. Let stand for 30 minutes

to drain.

Step 3

Preheat the oven to 425°. Roll out dough

between 2 sheets of plastic wrap to an 11"

round. Remove the top layer of plastic

wrap. Invert dough onto pie dish. Carefully

peel off plastic wrap.

Step 4

Toss both cheeses in a medium bowl until

evenly incorporated. Reserve 1/4 cup of

cheese mixture. Whisk scallion,

mayonnaise, dill, vinegar, sugar, salt, and

pepper in a small bowl.

Step 5

Sprinkle cornmeal evenly over bottom of

crust, then top with 1/2 cup cheese

mixture. Arrange 1/3 of tomatoes over

cheese, overlapping as needed. Spread half

of the mayonnaise mixture (about 1/3 cup)

over. Repeat layering with 1 cup of cheese

mixture, 1/2 of remaining tomato slices,

and remaining mayonnaise mixture.

Sprinkle the remaining 1 cup cheese

mixture over the remaining tomato slices.

Sprinkle with reserved 1/4 cup cheese

mixture. Fold overhanging crust up and over

edges of tomato slices.

Step 6

Bake pie until crust is golden and cheese is

golden brown, 35-40 minutes (check crust

halfway and tent with foil if it's getting too dark). Let pie cool at least 1 hour and up to 3 hours before slicing and serving.

Step 7

Editor's note: This recipe reflects the change made to the amount of buttermilk in the crust.

Green Spaghetti

INGREDIENTS

- 4 large poblano peppers

- 1/4 c. packed cilantro leaves, plus more for garnish

- 1 small yellow onion, chopped

- 2 cloves garlic, chopped

- 2 tbsp. butter

- 1/4 c. low-sodium vegetable stock or

  water

- 1 lb. spaghetti

- 4 oz. cream cheese, cubed

- Kosher salt

- Freshly ground black pepper

DIRECTIONS

1. Turn broiler to high and line a

    medium baking sheet with foil. Place

    peppers on baking sheet and broil,

turning occasionally with tongs, until blackened on all sides.

2. Transfer chilis to a heat-proof bowl and cover with plastic wrap. Let peppers steam for 10 minutes, then remove plastic wrap and peel skins off peppers.

3. Remove stems and seeds and roughly chop peppers.

4. Combine peppers, cilantro, onion, and garlic into a food processor or blender and blend until smooth.

5. In a large skillet over medium heat, melt butter. Pour in pepper mixture, then stir in vegetable stock or water. Cook, stirring occasionally, until thickened slightly, 3 to 4 minutes.

6. Meanwhile, make spaghetti: In a large pot of boiling salted water, cook spaghetti according to package instructions. Reserve 1 cup pasta water then drain.

7. Add cream cheese to sauce and stir until it has completely melted into the sauce. Season with salt and

pepper. Toss cooked pasta with sauce, adding pasta water to loosen up the sauce, if needed. Divide onto plates and garnish with cilantro and queso fresco.

Zucchini Tater Tots

INGREDIENTS

- cooking spray

- 3 large zucchini, grated

- 2 large eggs, lightly beaten

- 1/2 c. shredded cheddar

- 1/2 c. grated Parmesan

- 1 tsp. dried oregano

- 1/4 tsp. garlic powder

- 1/4 tsp. Kosher salt

- Freshly ground black pepper

- Ketchup, for serving

DIRECTIONS

1. Preheat the oven to 400°F and grease

   a baking sheet with cooking spray.

   Using a box grater, grate zucchini

   onto a clean kitchen towel. Gather

   ends of the kitchen towel to cover

   zucchini completely, then squeeze

   out excess liquid over the sink.

2. In a large bowl, whisk eggs until yokes

   are broken up and mixture is yellow.

   Add zucchini, cheddar, Parmesan,

   oregano,garlic powder, salt, and

   pepper and mix until combined.Scoop

   1 tablespoon of mixture and roll it

   into a tater-tot shape with your

   hands. Place on the baking sheet.

3. Bake until golden, 15 to 20 minutes.

   Serve with ketchup.

Appletoni

INGREDIENTS

- 1 1/2 oz. vodka

- 1 oz. apple schnapps

- 1/2 oz. calvados

- Ice

- Green apple slices, for serving

DIRECTIONS

1. Place the martini glass in the freezer

   to chill.

2. Combine vodka, schnapps, and

   calvados in a cocktail shaker. Fill with

   ice and shake until chilled, about 30

   seconds.

3. Pour cocktail into chilled glass and

    garnish with apple slices.

Avocado Pickles

INGREDIENTS

- 1 c. distilled white vinegar

- 1 c. water

- 1/3 c. sugar

- 1 tbsp. kosher salt

- 1 tsp. crushed red pepper flakes

- 1 clove garlic, thinly sliced

- 5 sprigs cilantro

- 2 underripe avocados, peeled and thinly sliced

DIRECTIONS

1. In a small saucepan over medium heat, combine vinegar, water, sugar and salt and bring to a boil, stirring frequently. When the sugar and salt have dissolved, set aside to cool.

2. In a mason jar, place red pepper flakes, garlic, cilantro, and avocado slices. Pour cooled pickling mixture into the jar and seal tightly with a lid.

3. Refrigerate for at least 3 hours before

    serving.

Broccoli Pesto

INGREDIENTS

- 1 head broccoli, florets removed and

  blanched

- 1 c. fresh basil leaves

- 1/2 c. extra-virgin olive oil

- 1/4 c. freshly grated Parmesan

- 1/4 c. almonds

- 1 clove garlic, minced

- 1 tsp. kosher salt

DIRECTIONS

1. In the bowl of a food processor, combine broccoli, basil, and oil and pulse until combined.

2. Add Parmesan, almonds, garlic, and salt and blend until combined.

3. Store in an airtight container for up to 1 week.

Avocado Cheesecake

INGREDIENTS

FOR THE CRUST

- 10 graham crackers

* 1/3 c. granulated sugar

* 6 tbsp. butter, melted

* kosher salt

FOR THE FILLING

* 2 8-oz blocks cream cheese, softened

* 2 ripe avocados, peeled and pitted

* 1 c. sugar

* Pinch salt

* 3/4 c. heavy cream

* 1/2 c. fresh lime juice

* Zest of 1 lime

* small lime wedges (for garnish)

DIRECTIONS

1. Preheat the oven to 350° and spray a pie dish with nonstick cooking spray.

Make crust

1. In a food processor, pulse graham crackers until fine crumbs form.

2. Transfer to a medium bowl then add melted butter, sugar, and a pinch of salt and mix until combined.

3. Press the graham cracker mixture firmly into the prepared dish. Bake until the crust looks slightly toasted, 8

to 10 minutes. Let cool to room

temperature.

Make filling

1. In a large bowl using a hand mixer or

    a stand mixer with the paddle

    attachment, beat cream cheese,

    sugar and a pinch of salt until smooth

    and fluffy, 3 minutes. Add avocados

    and beat until smooth.

2. Add heavy cream, lime juice, and

    most of the lime zest (save some for

    garnish!). Beat until stiff peaks form,

    2 to 3 minutes more.

3. Transfer filling to cooled pie crust.
    Garnish with more lime zest and
    small lime wedges. Freeze until solid,
    4 to 5 hours. Serve immediately.

Sunchoke and Cauliflower Soup

Ingredients

- 2 tablespoons unsalted butter, plus 2
  teaspoons softened butter

- 1 small celery rib, minced

- 1/2 small onion, minced

- 2 cups chicken stock or low-sodium
  broth

- 3/4 cup whole milk

- 1 pound cauliflower, cut into 1-inch florets

- 6 ounces sunchokes, peeled and cut into 1-inch pieces

- 1 thyme sprig

- 1 small garlic clove, minced

- Salt

- Four 1/4-inch-thick baguette slices, cut on the bias

- 1 tablespoon freshly grated Parmigiano-Reggiano cheese

- Freshly ground pepper

- 1/2 cup sunflower sprouts

Instructions

Step 1

In a large saucepan, melt the 2 tablespoons of butter. Add the celery and onion and cook over low heat until softened, about 6 minutes. Add the stock and milk and bring to a simmer over high heat. Add the cauliflower, sunchokes and thyme and bring to a boil. Simmer over low heat until the sunchokes are very tender, about 30 minutes; discard the thyme sprig.

Step 2

Meanwhile, preheat the oven to 350°. In a small bowl, mix the 2 teaspoons of softened butter with the garlic and season with salt. Spread the garlic butter on the baguette slices and place on a baking sheet. Sprinkle with the cheese and bake for about 8 minutes, until crisp.

Step 3

Working in batches, puree the soup in a blender until smooth. Return the soup to the saucepan; season with salt and pepper.

Ladle into bowls and top with the sprouts.

Serve with the cheese toasts.

Make Ahead

The sunchoke-cauliflower soup can be

refrigerated overnight.

Buttered Cauliflower Puree

Ingredients

- Two 2-pound heads of cauliflower,

    cored and separated into 2-inch

    florets

- 2 cups heavy cream

- 1 1/2 sticks unsalted butter

- Salt

- Cayenne pepper

Instructions

Step 1

Preheat the oven to 325°. In a large pot of boiling salted water, cook the cauliflower florets until tender, about 7 minutes. Drain well. Spread the cauliflower on a large rimmed baking sheet. Bake for about 5 minutes, to dry it out.

Step 2

In a small saucepan, combine the heavy cream with the butter and bring to a simmer over moderate heat just until the butter is melted.

Step 3

Working in batches, puree the cauliflower in a blender with the warm cream mixture; transfer the puree to a medium microwave-safe bowl. Season with salt and cayenne. Just before serving, reheat the puree in the microwave in 1-minute intervals, stirring occasionally.

Make Ahead

The cauliflower puree can be refrigerated

overnight and reheated in a microwave; stir

occasionally.

Rice Noodle Salad

Ingredients

- 4 scallions, white and light green

  parts thinly sliced, dark greens

  reserved

- 3 lemongrass stalks, smashed with

  the flat side of a knife

- 1/4 cup minced fresh ginger

- 1/2 cup Asian fish sauce

- 1 1/2 pounds boneless, skinless

  chicken breasts, halved lengthwise

- 2 serrano chiles, seeded and thinly

  sliced

- 1 large garlic clove, minced

- 1 tablespoon sugar

- 1/4 cup mirin

- 1/4 cup rice vinegar

- 1 pound pad thai rice noodles

- 1 small jicama (about 1 pound),

  peeled and cut into fine matchsticks

- 1/4 pound mung bean sprouts

- Peanuts, cilantro and lime wedges,

  for serving

Instructions

Step 1

In a soup pot, combine the dark scallion

greens with the lemongrass, 2 tablespoons

of the ginger and 2 tablespoons of the fish

sauce. Add 8 cups of water and bring to a

boil. Simmer for 20 minutes. Add the

chicken and simmer over low heat just until

cooked, about 10 minutes. Remove the

chicken. Strain the liquid into a heatproof

bowl and let cool. Shred the chicken, add it

to the liquid and refrigerate overnight.

Step 2

In a small bowl, combine the chiles, garlic,

sugar, mirin and vinegar with the remaining

2 tablespoons of ginger and 6 tablespoons

of fish sauce. Refrigerate overnight.

Step 3

Bring a large pot of water to a boil. Cook the

noodles until al dente, about 6 minutes.

Drain and cool under running water. Cut

into 6-inch lengths and pat dry, shaking the

colander occasionally. Transfer the noodles

to a bowl along with the jicama, bean

sprouts, sliced scallions and the dressing.

Drain the chicken and add it to the salad.

Serve with peanuts, cilantro and lime

wedges.

Make Ahead

The chicken and dressing can be

refrigerated overnight.

White Anchovy and Crisp Pita Bread Salad

Ingredients

- 12 marinated white anchovies, cut into 1-inch pieces

- Two 6-inch pita breads, split into 4 rounds

- 4 tablespoons unsalted butter, softened

- 1 medium shallot, thinly sliced and separated into rings

- 1 1/2 tablespoons white balsamic vinegar or balsamic vinegar

- 1 tablespoon extra-virgin olive oil

- 3/4 cup sour cream

- 1 garlic clove, minced

- Salt and freshly ground white pepper

- 2 large Belgian endives, cored and

  sliced crosswise 1/2 inch thick

Instructions

Step 1

Preheat the oven to 350°. Arrange the pitas

on a baking sheet, rough sides up, and

spread each round with 1 tablespoon of the

butter. Bake for about 8 minutes, until

crisp. Let cool and break into large pieces.

Step 2

Meanwhile, in a small bowl, steep the

shallot in the vinegar for 5 minutes. Stir in

the olive oil, then add the sour cream and

garlic and season with salt and pepper.

Step 3

In a large bowl, toss the endives with the

anchovies and toasted pita. Add the sour

cream dressing and toss well. Spoon onto 4

plates and serve.

Ingredients

- 500ml whole milk

- 1 onion, halved

- 1 bay leaf

- 2 cloves

- 50g butter

- 50g plain flour

Method

STEP 1

Gently bring 500ml whole milk to the boil in

a small saucepan with 1 halved onion,

studded with 1 bay leaf and 2 cloves. Turn

off the heat and leave to infuse for 20 mins.

STEP 2

Melt 50g butter in another saucepan, then

add 50g plain flour. Stir continuously until a

paste forms – this is called a roux. Continue

cooking for 2 mins.

STEP 3

Remove the onion, bay and cloves from the

milk with a slotted spoon and discard. Add

the infused milk to the roux gradually,

stirring as you go, until you get a smooth

sauce. Cook for 5-10 mins, stirring

continuously, until the sauce has thickened.

Season to taste.

Yellow Squash Casserole

Ingredients

- 4 cups yellow squash (sliced)

- 1/2 cup onion (diced)

- 2 tablespoons water

- 1 cracker (buttered, round, crushed)

- 1 cup shredded cheddar cheese

- 2 eggs (beaten)

- 3/4 cup milk

- 1/4 cup butter (melted)

- 1 teaspoon salt

- 1/4 teaspoon black pepper

- 2 tablespoons butter

Instructions

1. Preheat oven to 350*F

2. In a deep 12 inch skillet, add squash, onion & water.

3. Cook over medium heat just until pan is hot.

4. Place lid on and lower heat to medium low. Cook for 5 minutes with lid on until squash is tender.

5. Add half the crushed cracker rounds

    and half the cheese to squash and

    mix well.

6. Add eggs, milk, butter, salt & pepper

    and mix well.

7. Top mixture with remaining cracker

    crumbs and cheese.

8. Dot top of casserole with butter.

9. Bake for 25 minutes then devour!

Ingredients

- 2 1/3 cups Gold Medal All Purpose

  Flour

- 2 1/2 teaspoons baking powder

- 1/2 teaspoon salt

- 1 cup butter (or margarine, softened)

- 1 1/4 cups sugar

- 3 eggs

- 1 teaspoon vanilla

- 2/3 cup milk

Steps

1. Heat oven to 350°F. Place a paper
    baking cup in each of 24 regular-size
    muffin cups, grease bottoms and
    sides of muffin cups with shortening
    and lightly flour, or spray with baking
    spray with flour.

2. In a medium bowl, mix flour, baking
    powder and salt; set aside.

3. In a large bowl, beat butter with an
    electric mixer on medium speed for
    30 seconds. Gradually add sugar,
    about 1/4 cup at a time, beating well

after each addition and scraping the

bowl occasionally. Beat 2 minutes

longer. Add eggs, one at a time,

beating well after each addition. Beat

in vanilla. On low speed, alternately

add flour mixture, about one-third at

a time, and milk, about half at a time,

beating just until blended.

4. Divide batter evenly among muffin

cups, filling each with about 3

tablespoons of batter or until about

two-thirds full.

5. Bake 20 to 25 minutes or until a toothpick inserted in the center comes out clean. Cool for 5 minutes. Remove cupcakes from pans; place on cooling racks. Cool completely, about 30 minutes. Frost with desired frosting.

Thai Yellow Curry

Ingredients

- 1 small to medium carrots - chopped

- 8 to 10 baby corn - chopped

- 5 to 6 button mushrooms - chopped

- 1 small to medium red bell pepper - chopped (capsicum)

- 10 to 12 thai brinjals (baingan or eggplant)

- 1 cup thick coconut milk

- ½ teaspoon organic sugar

- 1 tablespoon chopped thai basil

- 1 or 2 teaspoon soy sauce

- to 2 cups water or veg stock

- 2 tablespoon coconut oil or vegetable oil

- a few thai basil leaves for garnish

- salt as required

For The Yellow Curry Paste

- 1 small onion or 1 to 2 shallots -

chopped

- 2 teaspoon coriander seeds

- 2 teaspoon cumin seeds or ground

cumin

- ¼ teaspoon black pepper

- 1 teaspoon ground turmeric or

turmeric powder (1 teaspoon gives a

dark yellow color, whereas you can

go for ½ teaspoon which will give a

light yellow color)

- 2 fresh thai red chillies or bird eyes chilies - chopped

- ½ inch galangal - chopped, substitute ginger if you don't have galangal

- 2 to 3 medium garlic cloves (lahsun) - roughly chopped

- 2 tablespoon coconut milk

- 2 medium kaffir lime leaves - roughly chopped (substitute ½ teaspoon of lemon zest)

- 1 stalk of lemongrass - chopped (skip if not available)

- ½ teaspoon lemon zest - optional

Instructions

Preparing Thai Yellow Curry Paste

1. Add all the ingredients for the paste in a chutney grinder or a small blender.

2. Blitz to make a smooth paste. I prefer to make a smooth paste so that the galangal and lemongrass bits and pieces don't come in the way while eating

3. Keep the curry paste aside.

Making Thai Yellow Curry

1. In a pot or pan, heat oil. add all of the yellow curry paste in oil and saute for 2 to 3 mins.

2. Then add 1/2 cup coconut milk and saute for 2 to 3 mins.

3. Then add the chopped veggies and stir well.

4. Add 1.5 to 2 cups water or veg stock, sugar and salt. stir well and cover the pan.

5. Simmer the veggies till they are almost cooked and tender.

6. Then add the remaining 1/2 cup
   coconut milk.

7. Stir and add soy sauce. cover and
   cook for about 5 to 6 minutes more.

8. Lastly add the chopped basil leaves
   and cook for half or one minute
   more.

9. You can garnish the curry with some
   thai basil leaves.

10.Serve thai yellow curry with steamed
   jasmine rice or basmati rice.

Notes

*substitutes for the thai herbs:

- galangal: use ginger instead

- kaffir lime leaves: add lime leaves or zest

of lemon instead

- thai chilies: substitute fresh red chilies or

dry red chilies

- shallots: use small onions instead

- lemon grass: no substitute. At the most,

you could just do away with the zest of

lemon

- thai basil: use italian basil as a substitute.

Purple Sweet Potato Collard Wraps

Ingredients

For the wraps

- 3-4 purple sweet potatoes

- 6 large collard leaves

- 3/4 tsp chili powder

- 1/4 tsp garlic powder

- red pepper flakes (optional)

- salt/pepper

- olive oil

- 2 large carrots, shredded

- sliced red onion

- sprouts

- roasted red pepper, sliced

- 1-2 ripe avocados, sliced

- chopped cashews

For the cashew honey mustard

- 1 cup cashews (preferably soaked for

  several hours prior)

- 1 tbs light olive oil

  - tbs yellow mustard

- 1 tbs honey

- 1 tsp apple cider vinegar

- 1/2 tsp ground ginger

- salt to taste

- water to thin

Instructions

1. Bring a pot of salted water to a boil.
   While waiting, peel and cube sweet
   potatoes. Add to water, reduce heat
   slightly and boil for 12-15 minutes,
   until soft.

2. While potatoes boil, add cashews,
   honey, mustard, light olive oil,
   vinegar, and ground ginger to a food
   processor. Pulse, adding water until
   you have a smooth sauce. Salt to
   taste.

3. Drain sweet potatoes and add salt,
    pepper, chili powder, garlic powder,
    and olive oil. Mash and add more oil
    as needed.

4. Wash collard leaves under very hot
    water (this will help them be a little
    bit malleable) Using a small paring
    knife, trim the thick vein that runs
    down the center of the leaf to make
    it lay flush with the rest of the leaf
    (careful not to pierce the leaf) Then
    cut the stem where the leaf starts.

5. Working one wrap at a time, lay collard leaf with the inside of the leaf facing up and the stem facing towards you. Spread a base of sweet potato mash, followed by a sprinkling of chopped cashews. Next, add your shredded carrots, roasted red pepper strips, and avocado slices. Top with sprouts.

6. Fold the right and left sides of the leaf inwards, then begin to roll your collard leaf, keeping it tight and tucking in the edges as you go. Secure

with two toothpicks and slice down

the center.

7. Repeat for the remaining wraps and

serve with cashew honey mustard.

Notes

You can make the wraps more pliable by

quickly dipping them into a pot of hot water

and then running the leaves under cold

water. I like to add crushed red pepper to

my wrap, as the extra kick compliments the

sweetness of the honey mustard. Leave that

out if you don't care for the extra kick. This

recipe makes enough for each person to have 1.5 wraps.

Purple Cauliflower Tabbouleh

Ingredients

- Tabbouleh

- 1 Head Purple Cauliflower

- 1/4 Red Onion diced

- 1 1/2 Cups Parsley packed, minced

- Hemp Seeds for Garnish

- Vinaigrette

- Juice from 1/2 Orange

- Juice from 1 Lemon

- 2 Tbs Extra Virgin Olive Oil

- 1 Tsp Salt

- 1 Tsp Pepper

- Zest of 1/2 Orange

Instructions

Tabbouleh

1. Start by making the cauliflower "rice". Cut the cauliflower into florets, and process in the food processor until a rice is formed. Be careful not to over-process!

2. Cut the red onion and mince the
    parsley, then fold into cauliflower
    rice. Set aside while you make the
    vinaigrette.

3. Vinaigrette

4. To make the dressing, combine all
    ingredients in a bowl and whisk until
    evenly combined. Add into tabbouleh
    and mix well.

5. Putting It All Together

6. Serve in bowls, garnished with hemp

    seeds and extra minced parsley.

7. Enjoy!

www.ingramcontent.com/pod-product-compliance
Lightning Source LLC
Chambersburg PA
CBHW050729260726
48661CB00001B/146